FIBROID-SHRINKING COOKBOOK

Delicious and Nutritious Meals for Supporting Women's Health and Well-Being

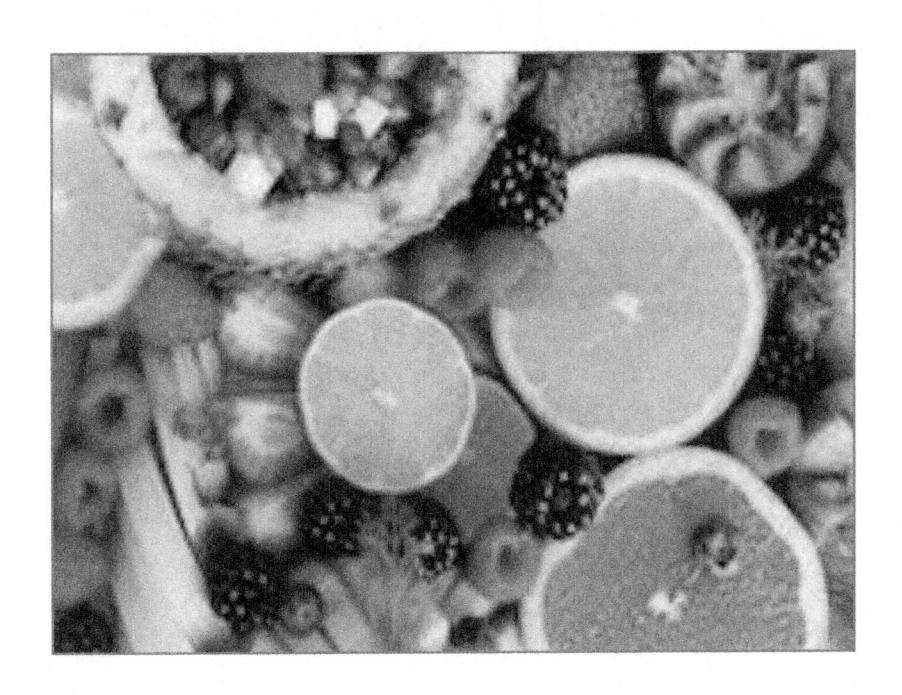

LAUREN WILLS

Copyright © 2023 Lauren Wills

All rights reserved. No part of this publication may be reproduced, distributed, or transmitted in any form or by any means, including photocopying, recording, or other electronic or mechanical methods, without the prior written permission of the publisher, except in the case of brief quotations embodied in critical reviews and certain other noncommercial uses permitted by copyright law.

This cookbook is intended for personal use only. It is protected by copyright laws and international treaties. Unauthorized reproduction or distribution of this work, or any portion thereof, may result in severe civil and criminal penalties, and will be prosecuted to the maximum extent possible under the law.

While every effort has been made to ensure the accuracy of the information presented in this cookbook, the author and the publisher cannot be held responsible for any errors, omissions, or damages arising out of the use of this cookbook. The recipes, cooking techniques, and nutritional information provided are for general informational purposes only and should not be considered a substitute for professional advice.

CONTENTS

CONTENTS 3

INTRODUCTION 6

FIBROID-SHRINKING RECIPES 8

   Recipe 1: Turmeric-Ginger Smoothie 8

   Recipe 2: Spinach and Kale Salad 9

   Recipe 3: Quinoa and Vegetable Stir-Fry 10

   Recipe 4: Lemon Garlic Shrimp 12

   Recipe 5: Berry Blast Smoothie 13

   Recipe 6: Sweet Potato and Chickpea Curry 14

   Recipe 7: Grilled Vegetable Skewers 16

   Recipe 8: Lentil and Vegetable Soup 17

   Recipe 9: Baked Salmon with Asparagus 19

   Recipe 10: Avocado and Cucumber Salad 20

   Recipe 11: Butternut Squash Soup 22

   Recipe 12: Broccoli and Cauliflower Bake 23

   Recipe 13: Chickpea and Spinach Curry 25

   Recipe 14: Berry Chia Pudding 26

   Recipe 15: Lemon Garlic Quinoa Salad 28

   Recipe 16: Stuffed Bell Peppers 29

Recipe 17: Greek Salad with Tzatziki Dressing 31

Recipe 18: Roasted Brussels Sprouts 32

Recipe 19: Lemon Herb Grilled Chicken 34

Recipe 20: Cabbage and Carrot Slaw 35

Recipe 21: Roasted Eggplant and Tomato Pasta 37

Recipe 22: Mango Avocado Salsa 39

Recipe 23: Mushroom and Spinach Stuffed Chicken Breast 40

Recipe 24: Blueberry Oatmeal Muffins 42

Recipe 25: Lemon-Honey Grilled Shrimp Skewers 44

Recipe 26: Balsamic Roasted Brussels Sprouts 45

Recipe 27: Paprika-Roasted Carrots 47

Recipe 28: Teriyaki Salmon 48

Recipe 29: Spaghetti Squash with Pesto 49

Recipe 30: Lemon Herb Quinoa Salad 51

Recipe 31: Cilantro-Lime Black Bean Salad 52

Recipe 32: Broccoli and White Bean Soup 53

Recipe 33: Spinach and Feta Stuffed Chicken Breast 55

Recipe 34: Quinoa and Black Bean Stuffed Peppers 56

Recipe 35: Greek Quinoa Salad 58

Fibroid-Shrinking Recipes cookbook

Recipe 36: Zucchini Noodles with Pesto............................60

Recipe 37: Roasted Sweet Potatoes with Cinnamon 61

Recipe 38: Strawberry Spinach Salad................................62

Recipe 39: Honey-Garlic Shrimp and Broccoli 63

Recipe 40: Quinoa and Chickpea Stuffed Bell Peppers.... 65

Recipe 41: Mediterranean Orzo Salad 67

Recipe 42: Grilled Lemon Garlic Asparagus.....................68

Recipe 43: Avocado Tomato Salad..................................... 69

Recipe 44: Butternut Squash and Apple Soup 71

Recipe 45: Baked Lemon Herb Tilapia 72

Recipe 46: Spinach and Mushroom Stuffed Acorn Squash 74

Recipe 47: Lemon Rosemary Grilled Chicken 75

Recipe 48: Roasted Beet and Goat Cheese Salad 77

Recipe 49: Quinoa-Stuffed Portobello Mushrooms 78

Recipe 50: Grilled Vegetable Platter with Hummus 80

CONCLUSION 82

INTRODUCTION

Welcome to the "Fibroid-Shrinking Recipes Cookbook," a collection of wholesome and delectable dishes designed to support women's health and well-being. This cookbook is not just a compilation of recipes; it's a journey towards better health and vitality.

Fibroids, noncancerous growths in the uterus, can be a source of discomfort and concern for many women. While medical treatments are available, a well-balanced diet filled with nutrient-rich foods can play a significant role in managing fibroids and promoting overall health. This cookbook aims to provide you with a variety of delicious and nutritious recipes that can aid in shrinking fibroids or alleviating related symptoms.

Each recipe in this cookbook is carefully crafted to incorporate ingredients that are known for their potential to support uterine health and hormonal balance. You'll find an array of dishes featuring fresh fruits and vegetables, lean proteins, whole grains, and herbs and spices that may contribute to your well-being.

Whether you're looking to actively manage fibroids or simply seeking a healthier lifestyle, these recipes offer a delicious way to nourish your body. From vibrant salads to comforting soups, hearty main courses to refreshing smoothies, and delightful desserts to energizing snacks, there's something here to satisfy every palate and dietary preference.

Remember, the journey to better health is not just about what you eat but also how you feel about what you're eating. Preparing and savoring these meals can be an act of self-care, promoting a sense of empowerment and wellness.

So, embark on this culinary adventure with us as we explore the intersection of flavor and health. Let these Fibroid-Shrinking Recipes be your guide to nurturing your body, supporting your well-being, and enjoying the delicious flavors of a balanced and wholesome diet. Here's to your health, vitality, and the joy of discovering how good food can be both a pleasure and a path to wellness.

FIBROID-SHRINKING RECIPES

Recipe 1: Turmeric-Ginger Smoothie

Prep Time: 5 minutes Serves: 1

Ingredients:

- 1 cup almond milk
- 1 ripe banana
- 1 tsp turmeric powder
- 1 tsp grated ginger
- 1/2 tsp cinnamon
- 1 tbsp honey
- 1/2 cup frozen pineapple chunks

Directions:

1. Place all ingredients in a blender.
2. Blend until smooth.
3. Pour into a glass and enjoy!

Nutritional Value:

- Calories: 245
- Protein: 2g

- Carbohydrates: 60g
- Fiber: 7g
- Fat: 1g

Recipe 2: Spinach and Kale Salad

Prep Time: 15 minutes Serves: 2

Ingredients:

- 2 cups fresh spinach leaves
- 2 cups fresh kale leaves, chopped
- 1/2 cup shredded carrots
- 1/4 cup sliced almonds
- 1/4 cup dried cranberries
- 2 tbsp olive oil
- 1 tbsp lemon juice
- Salt and pepper to taste

Directions:

1. In a large bowl, combine spinach, kale, carrots, almonds, and cranberries.

2. In a small bowl, whisk together olive oil, lemon juice, salt, and pepper.

3. Drizzle the dressing over the salad and toss well.

4. Serve and enjoy!

Nutritional Value:

- Calories: 236
- Protein: 6g
- Carbohydrates: 23g
- Fiber: 6g
- Fat: 15g

Recipe 3: Quinoa and Vegetable Stir-Fry

Prep Time: 20 minutes Serves: 4

Ingredients:

- 1 cup quinoa, cooked
- 1 cup broccoli florets
- 1 cup sliced bell peppers (red, yellow, or green)
- 1 cup sliced zucchini
- 1/2 cup sliced mushrooms

- 2 cloves garlic, minced
- 2 tbsp low-sodium soy sauce
- 1 tbsp sesame oil
- 1 tsp ginger, grated
- 1/4 tsp red pepper flakes (optional)

Directions:

1. In a large pan, heat sesame oil over medium heat.
2. Add minced garlic and grated ginger; sauté for 1 minute.
3. Add broccoli, bell peppers, zucchini, and mushrooms. Stir-fry for 5-7 minutes until vegetables are tender.
4. Add cooked quinoa, soy sauce, and red pepper flakes (if desired). Stir-fry for an additional 2 minutes.
5. Serve hot.

Nutritional Value:

- Calories: 210
- Protein: 8g
- Carbohydrates: 36g

- Fiber: 5g
- Fat: 4g

Recipe 4: Lemon Garlic Shrimp

Prep Time: 10 minutes Serves: 2

Ingredients:

- 12 large shrimp, peeled and deveined
- 2 cloves garlic, minced
- Zest and juice of 1 lemon
- 1 tbsp olive oil
- 1/4 tsp salt
- 1/4 tsp black pepper
- 1/2 tsp dried oregano
- Fresh parsley for garnish

Directions:

1. In a bowl, combine minced garlic, lemon zest, lemon juice, olive oil, salt, black pepper, and oregano.
2. Toss the shrimp in the marinade and let it sit for 5 minutes.

3. Heat a skillet over medium-high heat and add the marinated shrimp.

4. Cook for 2-3 minutes per side until pink and opaque.

5. Garnish with fresh parsley and serve.

Nutritional Value:

- Calories: 147
- Protein: 18g
- Carbohydrates: 3g
- Fiber: 0g
- Fat: 7g

Recipe 5: Berry Blast Smoothie

Prep Time: 5 minutes Serves: 1

Ingredients:

- 1 cup mixed berries (strawberries, blueberries, raspberries)
- 1/2 cup Greek yogurt
- 1/2 cup unsweetened almond milk
- 1 tbsp honey

- 1/2 tsp vanilla extract
- 1/4 cup rolled oats

Directions:

1. Place all ingredients in a blender.
2. Blend until smooth and creamy.
3. Pour into a glass and enjoy!

Nutritional Value:

- Calories: 278
- Protein: 13g
- Carbohydrates: 53g
- Fiber: 9g
- Fat: 4g

Recipe 6: Sweet Potato and Chickpea Curry

Prep Time: 30 minutes Serves: 4

Ingredients:

- 2 sweet potatoes, peeled and diced
- 1 can (15 oz) chickpeas, drained and rinsed
- 1 onion, chopped

- 2 cloves garlic, minced
- 1 can (14 oz) diced tomatoes
- 1 can (14 oz) coconut milk
- 2 tsp curry powder
- 1 tsp ground cumin
- 1/2 tsp ground coriander
- Salt and pepper to taste
- Fresh cilantro for garnish

Directions:

1. In a large pot, sauté onions and garlic in a bit of oil until translucent.
2. Add curry powder, cumin, and coriander. Stir for 1 minute.
3. Add sweet potatoes, chickpeas, diced tomatoes, and coconut milk. Season with salt and pepper.
4. Simmer for 20 minutes or until sweet potatoes are tender.
5. Garnish with fresh cilantro and serve over rice or quinoa.

Nutritional Value:

- Calories: 347
- Protein: 8g
- Carbohydrates: 49g
- Fiber: 10g
- Fat: 16g

Recipe 7: Grilled Vegetable Skewers

Prep Time: 15 minutes Cook Time: 10 minutes Serves: 4

Ingredients:

- 2 zucchinis, cut into rounds
- 1 red onion, cut into chunks
- 1 red bell pepper, cut into chunks
- 1 yellow bell pepper, cut into chunks
- 1/4 cup olive oil
- 2 cloves garlic, minced
- 1 tsp dried oregano
- 1/2 tsp salt
- 1/4 tsp black pepper

Directions:

1. Preheat the grill to medium-high heat.
2. In a bowl, combine olive oil, minced garlic, oregano, salt, and black pepper.
3. Thread the vegetables onto skewers and brush with the olive oil mixture.
4. Grill for about 10 minutes, turning occasionally, until vegetables are tender and slightly charred.
5. Serve hot as a side dish or over quinoa for a complete meal.

Nutritional Value:

- Calories: 162
- Protein: 2g
- Carbohydrates: 13g
- Fiber: 4g
- Fat: 12g

Recipe 8: Lentil and Vegetable Soup

Prep Time: 15 minutes Cook Time: 30 minutes Serves: 6

Ingredients:

- 1 cup dried green or brown lentils, rinsed and drained
- 1 onion, chopped
- 2 carrots, peeled and chopped
- 2 celery stalks, chopped
- 2 cloves garlic, minced
- 1 can (14 oz) diced tomatoes
- 6 cups vegetable broth
- 1 tsp dried thyme
- 1 tsp paprika
- Salt and pepper to taste
- Fresh parsley for garnish

Directions:

1. In a large pot, sauté onions, carrots, celery, and garlic until softened.
2. Add lentils, diced tomatoes, vegetable broth, thyme, paprika, salt, and pepper.
3. Bring to a boil, then reduce heat and simmer for 25-30 minutes, or until lentils are tender.

4. Garnish with fresh parsley and serve.

Nutritional Value:

- Calories: 193
- Protein: 11g
- Carbohydrates: 34g
- Fiber: 13g
- Fat: 1g

Recipe 9: Baked Salmon with Asparagus

Prep Time: 15 minutes Cook Time: 20 minutes Serves: 2

Ingredients:

- 2 salmon fillets
- 1 bunch asparagus, trimmed
- 2 tbsp olive oil
- 2 cloves garlic, minced
- 1 tsp lemon zest
- 1 tbsp lemon juice
- Salt and pepper to taste
- Fresh dill for garnish

Directions:

1. Preheat the oven to 400°F (200°C).
2. Place salmon fillets and asparagus on a baking sheet.
3. In a small bowl, whisk together olive oil, minced garlic, lemon zest, lemon juice, salt, and pepper.
4. Drizzle the mixture over the salmon and asparagus.
5. Bake for 15-20 minutes, or until salmon flakes easily with a fork.
6. Garnish with fresh dill and serve.

Nutritional Value:

- Calories: 348
- Protein: 38g
- Carbohydrates: 6g
- Fiber: 3g
- Fat: 19g

Recipe 10: Avocado and Cucumber Salad

Prep Time: 10 minutes Serves: 2

Ingredients:

- 2 avocados, diced
- 1 cucumber, diced
- 1/4 red onion, thinly sliced
- 2 tbsp fresh lime juice
- 2 tbsp olive oil
- Salt and pepper to taste
- Fresh cilantro for garnish

Directions:

1. In a bowl, combine diced avocados, diced cucumber, and sliced red onion.
2. In a separate bowl, whisk together lime juice, olive oil, salt, and pepper.
3. Drizzle the dressing over the salad and toss gently.
4. Garnish with fresh cilantro and serve.

Nutritional Value:

- Calories: 275
- Protein: 3g
- Carbohydrates: 15g

- Fiber: 9g
- Fat: 24g

Recipe 11: Butternut Squash Soup

Prep Time: 20 minutes Cook Time: 30 minutes Serves: 4

Ingredients:

- 1 butternut squash, peeled and diced
- 1 onion, chopped
- 2 carrots, peeled and chopped
- 2 cloves garlic, minced
- 4 cups vegetable broth
- 1 tsp ground cumin
- 1/2 tsp ground cinnamon
- 1/4 tsp nutmeg
- Salt and pepper to taste
- Greek yogurt for garnish

Directions:

1. In a large pot, sauté onions, carrots, and garlic until softened.

2. Add butternut squash, vegetable broth, cumin, cinnamon, nutmeg, salt, and pepper.

3. Bring to a boil, then reduce heat and simmer for 25-30 minutes, or until squash is tender.

4. Use an immersion blender to puree the soup until smooth.

5. Serve hot with a dollop of Greek yogurt.

Nutritional Value:

- Calories: 184
- Protein: 3g
- Carbohydrates: 45g
- Fiber: 7g
- Fat: 1g

Recipe 12: Broccoli and Cauliflower Bake

Prep Time: 15 minutes Cook Time: 25 minutes Serves: 4

Ingredients:

- 2 cups broccoli florets
- 2 cups cauliflower florets
- 1/4 cup grated Parmesan cheese

- 1/4 cup Greek yogurt
- 1/4 cup shredded cheddar cheese
- 1/4 tsp garlic powder
- Salt and pepper to taste

Directions:

1. Steam broccoli and cauliflower until tender-crisp.
2. In a bowl, mix together grated Parmesan cheese, Greek yogurt, garlic powder, salt, and pepper.
3. Add steamed vegetables to the bowl and toss to coat.
4. Transfer the mixture to a baking dish and sprinkle with shredded cheddar cheese.
5. Bake at 375°F (190°C) for 20-25 minutes, or until cheese is bubbly and golden.
6. Serve as a side dish.

Nutritional Value:

- Calories: 123
- Protein: 9g
- Carbohydrates: 10g

- Fiber: 4g
- Fat: 6g

Recipe 13: Chickpea and Spinach Curry

Prep Time: 15 minutes Cook Time: 20 minutes Serves: 4

Ingredients:

- 2 cans (15 oz each) chickpeas, drained and rinsed
- 2 cups fresh spinach leaves
- 1 onion, chopped
- 2 cloves garlic, minced
- 1 can (14 oz) diced tomatoes
- 1 can (14 oz) coconut milk
- 2 tsp curry powder
- 1 tsp ground turmeric
- 1/2 tsp cayenne pepper (adjust to taste)
- Salt and pepper to taste
- Fresh cilantro for garnish

Directions:

1. In a large pan, sauté onions and garlic until softened.

2. Add chickpeas, diced tomatoes, coconut milk, curry powder, turmeric, cayenne pepper, salt, and pepper.

3. Simmer for 15-20 minutes, stirring occasionally.

4. Stir in fresh spinach and cook until wilted.

5. Garnish with fresh cilantro and serve over rice or quinoa.

Nutritional Value:

- Calories: 325
- Protein: 11g
- Carbohydrates: 46g
- Fiber: 12g
- Fat: 13g

Recipe 14: Berry Chia Pudding

Prep Time: 5 minutes Chill Time: 4 hours or overnight Serves: 2

Ingredients:

- 1/4 cup chia seeds
- 1 cup almond milk
- 1/2 tsp vanilla extract

- 1 cup mixed berries (strawberries, blueberries, raspberries)
- 1 tbsp honey (optional)

Directions:

1. In a bowl, mix chia seeds, almond milk, and vanilla extract.
2. Stir well, cover, and refrigerate for at least 4 hours or overnight.
3. Before serving, layer the chia pudding and mixed berries in serving glasses.
4. Drizzle with honey if desired.

Nutritional Value:

- Calories: 177
- Protein: 4g
- Carbohydrates: 27g
- Fiber: 10g
- Fat: 6g

Recipe 15: Lemon Garlic Quinoa Salad

Prep Time: 15 minutes Serves: 4

Ingredients:

- 1 cup quinoa, cooked and cooled
- 1 cucumber, diced
- 1 red bell pepper, diced
- 1/4 cup red onion, finely chopped
- 1/4 cup fresh parsley, chopped
- Zest and juice of 1 lemon
- 2 tbsp olive oil
- Salt and pepper to taste

Directions:

1. In a large bowl, combine quinoa, diced cucumber, diced red bell pepper, chopped red onion, and fresh parsley.
2. In a separate bowl, whisk together lemon zest, lemon juice, olive oil, salt, and pepper.
3. Drizzle the dressing over the salad and toss well.
4. Serve chilled.

Nutritional Value:

- Calories: 233
- Protein: 6g
- Carbohydrates: 35g
- Fiber: 5g
- Fat: 9g

Recipe 16: Stuffed Bell Peppers

Prep Time: 20 minutes Cook Time: 45 minutes Serves: 4

Ingredients:

- 4 large bell peppers, any color
- 1 cup cooked quinoa
- 1 cup black beans, drained and rinsed
- 1 cup diced tomatoes
- 1 cup corn kernels (fresh or frozen)
- 1/2 cup shredded cheddar cheese
- 1/2 tsp chili powder
- Salt and pepper to taste
- Fresh cilantro for garnish

Directions:

1. Preheat the oven to 375°F (190°C).
2. Cut the tops off the bell peppers and remove seeds and membranes.
3. In a bowl, mix cooked quinoa, black beans, diced tomatoes, corn, shredded cheddar cheese, chili powder, salt, and pepper.
4. Stuff each bell pepper with the quinoa mixture.
5. Place stuffed peppers in a baking dish and cover with foil.
6. Bake for 30 minutes, then remove foil and bake for an additional 15 minutes until peppers are tender and cheese is melted.
7. Garnish with fresh cilantro and serve.

Nutritional Value:

- Calories: 285
- Protein: 12g
- Carbohydrates: 49g
- Fiber: 11g

- Fat: 6g

Recipe 17: Greek Salad with Tzatziki Dressing

Prep Time: 15 minutes Serves: 4

Ingredients:

- 2 cups cucumber, diced
- 2 cups cherry tomatoes, halved
- 1/2 red onion, thinly sliced
- 1/2 cup Kalamata olives, pitted
- 1/2 cup crumbled feta cheese
- 2 tbsp fresh dill, chopped
- 1/4 cup plain Greek yogurt
- 1/4 cup sour cream
- 1 tbsp lemon juice
- 1 clove garlic, minced
- Salt and pepper to taste

Directions:

1. In a large bowl, combine diced cucumber, halved cherry tomatoes, sliced red onion, Kalamata olives, crumbled feta cheese, and fresh dill.

2. In a separate bowl, whisk together Greek yogurt, sour cream, lemon juice, minced garlic, salt, and pepper to make the tzatziki dressing.

3. Drizzle the dressing over the salad and toss gently.

4. Serve as a refreshing side dish.

Nutritional Value:

- Calories: 187
- Protein: 7g
- Carbohydrates: 13g
- Fiber: 3g
- Fat: 13g

Recipe 18: Roasted Brussels Sprouts

Prep Time: 10 minutes Cook Time: 25 minutes Serves: 4

Ingredients:

- 1 lb Brussels sprouts, trimmed and halved

- 2 tbsp olive oil
- 2 cloves garlic, minced
- 1/4 cup grated Parmesan cheese
- Salt and pepper to taste
- Lemon wedges for serving

Directions:

1. Preheat the oven to 400°F (200°C).
2. In a bowl, toss Brussels sprouts with olive oil and minced garlic.
3. Spread them out on a baking sheet in a single layer.
4. Roast for 20-25 minutes, stirring once, until sprouts are tender and browned.
5. Sprinkle with grated Parmesan cheese, salt, and pepper.
6. Serve with lemon wedges for extra flavor.

Nutritional Value:

- Calories: 126
- Protein: 5g

- Carbohydrates: 10g
- Fiber: 4g
- Fat: 8g

Recipe 19: Lemon Herb Grilled Chicken

Prep Time: 15 minutes Cook Time: 15 minutes Serves: 2

Ingredients:

- 2 boneless, skinless chicken breasts
- Zest and juice of 1 lemon
- 2 tbsp olive oil
- 2 cloves garlic, minced
- 1 tsp dried thyme
- 1 tsp dried rosemary
- Salt and pepper to taste
- Fresh parsley for garnish

Directions:

1. In a bowl, mix together lemon zest, lemon juice, olive oil, minced garlic, dried thyme, dried rosemary, salt, and pepper.

2. Marinate chicken breasts in the mixture for at least 15 minutes.

3. Preheat the grill to medium-high heat.

4. Grill chicken for about 6-7 minutes per side, or until cooked through.

5. Garnish with fresh parsley and serve.

Nutritional Value:

- Calories: 294
- Protein: 29g
- Carbohydrates: 3g
- Fiber: 1g
- Fat: 19g

Recipe 20: Cabbage and Carrot Slaw

Prep Time: 10 minutes Serves: 4

Ingredients:

- 4 cups shredded cabbage (green or purple)
- 1 cup shredded carrots
- 1/4 cup plain Greek yogurt

- 2 tbsp mayonnaise
- 1 tbsp apple cider vinegar
- 1 tbsp honey
- 1/2 tsp celery seeds
- Salt and pepper to taste

Directions:

1. In a large bowl, combine shredded cabbage and shredded carrots.
2. In a separate bowl, whisk together Greek yogurt, mayonnaise, apple cider vinegar, honey, celery seeds, salt, and pepper.
3. Pour the dressing over the cabbage and carrots, and toss until well coated.
4. Chill in the refrigerator for at least 30 minutes before serving.

Nutritional Value:

- Calories: 99
- Protein: 2g
- Carbohydrates: 15g

- Fiber: 3g
- Fat: 4g

Recipe 21: Roasted Eggplant and Tomato Pasta

Prep Time: 15 minutes Cook Time: 30 minutes Serves: 4

Ingredients:

- 1 eggplant, diced
- 2 cups cherry tomatoes
- 4 cloves garlic, minced
- 2 tbsp olive oil
- 1 tsp dried basil
- 1/2 tsp dried oregano
- Salt and pepper to taste
- 8 oz whole wheat pasta
- Fresh basil leaves for garnish
- Grated Parmesan cheese (optional)

Directions:

1. Preheat the oven to 400°F (200°C).

2. In a large bowl, toss diced eggplant, cherry tomatoes, minced garlic, olive oil, dried basil, dried oregano, salt, and pepper.

3. Spread the mixture on a baking sheet in a single layer.

4. Roast for 25-30 minutes, stirring occasionally, until vegetables are tender and slightly caramelized.

5. Meanwhile, cook pasta according to package instructions.

6. Toss the roasted vegetables with cooked pasta.

7. Garnish with fresh basil leaves and grated Parmesan cheese if desired.

Nutritional Value:

- Calories: 310
- Protein: 9g
- Carbohydrates: 55g
- Fiber: 9g
- Fat: 8g

Recipe 22: Mango Avocado Salsa

Prep Time: 10 minutes Serves: 4

Ingredients:

- 1 ripe mango, diced
- 1 ripe avocado, diced
- 1/4 cup red onion, finely chopped
- 1/4 cup fresh cilantro, chopped
- Juice of 1 lime
- Salt and pepper to taste
- Tortilla chips for serving

Directions:

1. In a bowl, combine diced mango, diced avocado, chopped red onion, and chopped fresh cilantro.
2. Squeeze the juice of one lime over the mixture.
3. Season with salt and pepper, and gently toss to combine.
4. Serve with tortilla chips as a delicious snack or appetizer.

Nutritional Value:

- Calories: 126
- Protein: 2g
- Carbohydrates: 16g
- Fiber: 5g
- Fat: 7g

Recipe 23: Mushroom and Spinach Stuffed Chicken Breast

Prep Time: 20 minutes Cook Time: 25 minutes Serves: 2

Ingredients:

- 2 boneless, skinless chicken breasts
- 1 cup mushrooms, finely chopped
- 1 cup fresh spinach, chopped
- 1/4 cup grated Parmesan cheese
- 2 cloves garlic, minced
- 1 tbsp olive oil
- Salt and pepper to taste
- Toothpicks or kitchen twine

Directions:

1. Preheat the oven to 375°F (190°C).

2. In a pan, heat olive oil over medium heat. Add minced garlic and sauté for 1 minute.

3. Add chopped mushrooms and spinach to the pan. Cook until spinach wilts and mushrooms release their moisture.

4. Remove from heat and stir in grated Parmesan cheese, salt, and pepper.

5. Carefully cut a pocket into each chicken breast.

6. Stuff each chicken breast with the mushroom and spinach mixture, securing with toothpicks or kitchen twine.

7. Place stuffed chicken breasts in a baking dish and bake for 20-25 minutes, or until chicken is cooked through.

8. Remove toothpicks or twine before serving.

Nutritional Value:

- Calories: 287
- Protein: 42g
- Carbohydrates: 4g

- Fiber: 1g
- Fat: 11g

Recipe 24: Blueberry Oatmeal Muffins

Prep Time: 15 minutes Cook Time: 20 minutes Makes: 12 muffins

Ingredients:

- 1 cup rolled oats
- 1 cup whole wheat flour
- 1/2 cup brown sugar
- 1 tsp baking powder
- 1/2 tsp baking soda
- 1/2 tsp cinnamon
- 1/4 tsp salt
- 1 cup plain Greek yogurt
- 2 eggs
- 1/4 cup unsweetened applesauce
- 1 tsp vanilla extract
- 1 cup blueberries (fresh or frozen)

Directions:

1. Preheat the oven to 350°F (175°C) and line a muffin tin with paper liners.
2. In a bowl, mix rolled oats, whole wheat flour, brown sugar, baking powder, baking soda, cinnamon, and salt.
3. In another bowl, whisk together Greek yogurt, eggs, applesauce, and vanilla extract.
4. Combine the wet and dry ingredients, then gently fold in the blueberries.
5. Divide the batter evenly among the muffin cups.
6. Bake for 18-20 minutes, or until a toothpick inserted into the center comes out clean.
7. Allow muffins to cool before serving.

Nutritional Value (per muffin):

- Calories: 125
- Protein: 5g
- Carbohydrates: 24g
- Fiber: 2g

- Fat: 2g

Recipe 25: Lemon-Honey Grilled Shrimp Skewers

Prep Time: 20 minutes Cook Time: 10 minutes Serves: 4

Ingredients:

- 16 large shrimp, peeled and deveined
- Zest and juice of 1 lemon
- 2 tbsp honey
- 2 tbsp olive oil
- 2 cloves garlic, minced
- 1/4 tsp red pepper flakes (adjust to taste)
- Salt and pepper to taste
- Wooden skewers, soaked in water for 30 minutes

Directions:

1. In a bowl, whisk together lemon zest, lemon juice, honey, olive oil, minced garlic, red pepper flakes, salt, and pepper.
2. Thread 4 shrimp onto each wooden skewer.
3. Brush the shrimp with the lemon-honey mixture.

4. Preheat the grill to medium-high heat and grill the shrimp skewers for about 2-3 minutes per side, or until pink and opaque.

5. Serve hot as a delicious appetizer or main dish.

Nutritional Value:

- Calories: 138
- Protein: 13g
- Carbohydrates: 8g
- Fiber: 0g
- Fat: 7g

Recipe 26: Balsamic Roasted Brussels Sprouts

Prep Time: 10 minutes Cook Time: 25 minutes Serves: 4

Ingredients:

- 1 lb Brussels sprouts, trimmed and halved
- 2 tbsp balsamic vinegar
- 2 tbsp olive oil
- 2 cloves garlic, minced
- Salt and pepper to taste

- Grated Parmesan cheese (optional)

Directions:

1. Preheat the oven to 400°F (200°C).
2. In a bowl, combine halved Brussels sprouts, balsamic vinegar, olive oil, minced garlic, salt, and pepper.
3. Spread them on a baking sheet in a single layer.
4. Roast for 20-25 minutes, stirring once, until sprouts are tender and caramelized.
5. Sprinkle with grated Parmesan cheese before serving if desired.

Nutritional Value:

- Calories: 124
- Protein: 4g
- Carbohydrates: 11g
- Fiber: 4g
- Fat: 8g

Recipe 27: Paprika-Roasted Carrots

Prep Time: 10 minutes Cook Time: 20 minutes Serves: 4

Ingredients:

- 4 large carrots, peeled and cut into sticks
- 2 tbsp olive oil
- 1 tsp paprika
- Salt and pepper to taste
- Fresh parsley for garnish

Directions:

1. Preheat the oven to 425°F (220°C).
2. In a bowl, toss carrot sticks with olive oil, paprika, salt, and pepper.
3. Spread them on a baking sheet in a single layer.
4. Roast for 15-20 minutes, stirring once, until carrots are tender and slightly caramelized.
5. Garnish with fresh parsley and serve.

Nutritional Value:

- Calories: 87

- Protein: 1g
- Carbohydrates: 8g
- Fiber: 2g
- Fat: 6g

Recipe 28: Teriyaki Salmon

Prep Time: 15 minutes Cook Time: 15 minutes Serves: 2

Ingredients:

- 2 salmon fillets
- 1/4 cup low-sodium teriyaki sauce
- 2 tbsp honey
- 1 tbsp rice vinegar
- 1 clove garlic, minced
- 1 tsp grated ginger
- Sesame seeds for garnish
- Sliced green onions for garnish

Directions:

1. In a bowl, whisk together teriyaki sauce, honey, rice vinegar, minced garlic, and grated ginger.

2. Marinate salmon fillets in the mixture for 10 minutes.

3. Preheat the grill to medium-high heat.

4. Grill salmon for about 6-7 minutes per side, or until cooked through.

5. Garnish with sesame seeds and sliced green onions before serving.

Nutritional Value:

- Calories: 321
- Protein: 35g
- Carbohydrates: 22g
- Fiber: 0g
- Fat: 12g

Recipe 29: Spaghetti Squash with Pesto

Prep Time: 10 minutes Cook Time: 40 minutes Serves: 4

Ingredients:

- 1 spaghetti squash, halved and seeds removed
- 2 tbsp olive oil
- 1/4 cup basil pesto

- 1/4 cup grated Parmesan cheese
- Salt and pepper to taste
- Fresh basil leaves for garnish

Directions:

1. Preheat the oven to 375°F (190°C).
2. Brush the cut sides of the spaghetti squash with olive oil and season with salt and pepper.
3. Place squash halves, cut side down, on a baking sheet.
4. Roast for 35-40 minutes until the flesh is tender and easily scraped with a fork.
5. Scrape the spaghetti-like strands of squash with a fork into a bowl.
6. Toss with basil pesto and grated Parmesan cheese.
7. Garnish with fresh basil leaves and serve.

Nutritional Value:

- Calories: 243
- Protein: 4g
- Carbohydrates: 14g

- Fiber: 3g
- Fat: 20g

Recipe 30: Lemon Herb Quinoa Salad

Prep Time: 15 minutes Serves: 4

Ingredients:

- 1 cup quinoa, cooked and cooled
- Zest and juice of 1 lemon
- 2 tbsp olive oil
- 1/4 cup fresh parsley, chopped
- 1/4 cup fresh mint, chopped
- 1/4 cup crumbled feta cheese
- Salt and pepper to taste
- Cherry tomatoes for garnish

Directions:

1. In a bowl, mix cooked quinoa, lemon zest, lemon juice, olive oil, chopped parsley, chopped mint, crumbled feta cheese, salt, and pepper.
2. Serve chilled, garnished with cherry tomatoes.

Nutritional Value:

- Calories: 219
- Protein: 6g
- Carbohydrates: 27g
- Fiber: 4g
- Fat: 10g

Recipe 31: Cilantro-Lime Black Bean Salad

Prep Time: 10 minutes Serves: 4

Ingredients:

- 2 cans (15 oz each) black beans, drained and rinsed
- 1 cup corn kernels (fresh or frozen)
- 1/2 cup red bell pepper, diced
- 1/4 cup fresh cilantro, chopped
- Zest and juice of 1 lime
- 2 tbsp olive oil
- 1 clove garlic, minced
- Salt and pepper to taste
- Avocado slices for garnish

Directions:

1. In a large bowl, combine black beans, corn kernels, diced red bell pepper, chopped cilantro, lime zest, and lime juice.
2. In a separate bowl, whisk together olive oil, minced garlic, salt, and pepper.
3. Drizzle the dressing over the salad and toss gently.
4. Garnish with avocado slices and serve.

Nutritional Value:

- Calories: 273
- Protein: 10g
- Carbohydrates: 44g
- Fiber: 10g
- Fat: 8g

Recipe 32: Broccoli and White Bean Soup

Prep Time: 15 minutes Cook Time: 25 minutes Serves: 4

Ingredients:

- 2 cups broccoli florets
- 1 can (15 oz) cannellini beans, drained and rinsed

- 1 onion, chopped
- 2 cloves garlic, minced
- 4 cups vegetable broth
- 1 tsp dried thyme
- Salt and pepper to taste
- Grated Parmesan cheese for garnish (optional)

Directions:

1. In a large pot, sauté chopped onions and minced garlic until softened.
2. Add broccoli florets, cannellini beans, vegetable broth, dried thyme, salt, and pepper.
3. Bring to a boil, then reduce heat and simmer for 20-25 minutes, or until broccoli is tender.
4. Use an immersion blender to puree the soup until smooth.
5. Garnish with grated Parmesan cheese if desired.

Nutritional Value:

- Calories: 185
- Protein: 10g

- Carbohydrates: 33g
- Fiber: 8g
- Fat: 1g

Recipe 33: Spinach and Feta Stuffed Chicken Breast

Prep Time: 20 minutes Cook Time: 25 minutes Serves: 2

Ingredients:

- 2 boneless, skinless chicken breasts
- 2 cups fresh spinach leaves
- 1/4 cup crumbled feta cheese
- 2 cloves garlic, minced
- 1 tbsp olive oil
- Salt and pepper to taste
- Toothpicks or kitchen twine

Directions:

1. Preheat the oven to 375°F (190°C).
2. Heat olive oil in a pan over medium heat. Add minced garlic and sauté for 1 minute.
3. Add fresh spinach to the pan and cook until wilted.

4. Carefully cut a pocket into each chicken breast.

5. Stuff each chicken breast with the spinach and feta mixture, securing with toothpicks or kitchen twine.

6. Place stuffed chicken breasts in a baking dish and bake for 20-25 minutes, or until chicken is cooked through.

7. Remove toothpicks or twine before serving.

Nutritional Value:

- Calories: 281
- Protein: 42g
- Carbohydrates: 4g
- Fiber: 1g
- Fat: 11g

Recipe 34: Quinoa and Black Bean Stuffed Peppers

Prep Time: 20 minutes Cook Time: 45 minutes Serves: 4

Ingredients:

- 4 large bell peppers, any color
- 1 cup cooked quinoa
- 1 can (15 oz) black beans, drained and rinsed

- 1 cup diced tomatoes
- 1 cup corn kernels (fresh or frozen)
- 1/2 cup shredded cheddar cheese
- 1/2 tsp chili powder
- Salt and pepper to taste
- Fresh cilantro for garnish

Directions:

1. Preheat the oven to 375°F (190°C).
2. Cut the tops off the bell peppers and remove seeds and membranes.
3. In a bowl, mix cooked quinoa, black beans, diced tomatoes, corn, shredded cheddar cheese, chili powder, salt, and pepper.
4. Stuff each bell pepper with the quinoa mixture.
5. Place stuffed peppers in a baking dish and cover with foil.
6. Bake for 30 minutes, then remove foil and bake for an additional 15 minutes until peppers are tender and cheese is melted.

7. Garnish with fresh cilantro and serve.

Nutritional Value:

- Calories: 305
- Protein: 14g
- Carbohydrates: 49g
- Fiber: 12g
- Fat: 7g

Recipe 35: Greek Quinoa Salad

Prep Time: 15 minutes Serves: 4

Ingredients:

- 2 cups cooked quinoa, cooled
- 1 cup cucumber, diced
- 1 cup cherry tomatoes, halved
- 1/2 cup Kalamata olives, pitted and sliced
- 1/2 cup crumbled feta cheese
- 1/4 cup red onion, thinly sliced
- 2 tbsp fresh dill, chopped
- Juice of 1 lemon

- 2 tbsp olive oil
- Salt and pepper to taste

Directions:

1. In a large bowl, combine cooked quinoa, diced cucumber, halved cherry tomatoes, sliced Kalamata olives, crumbled feta cheese, thinly sliced red onion, and chopped fresh dill.
2. In a separate bowl, whisk together lemon juice, olive oil, salt, and pepper.
3. Drizzle the dressing over the salad and toss gently.
4. Serve as a refreshing side dish.

Nutritional Value:

- Calories: 289
- Protein: 9g
- Carbohydrates: 33g
- Fiber: 5g
- Fat: 15g

Recipe 36: Zucchini Noodles with Pesto

Prep Time: 15 minutes Cook Time: 5 minutes Serves: 2

Ingredients:

- 2 large zucchinis, spiralized into noodles
- 1/4 cup basil pesto
- 1/4 cup cherry tomatoes, halved
- 1/4 cup pine nuts, toasted
- Grated Parmesan cheese for garnish (optional)
- Fresh basil leaves for garnish

Directions:

1. Heat a large skillet over medium heat.
2. Add spiralized zucchini noodles and cook for 3-5 minutes, tossing gently, until slightly softened.
3. Remove from heat and toss with basil pesto.
4. Garnish with cherry tomatoes, toasted pine nuts, grated Parmesan cheese, and fresh basil leaves before serving.

Nutritional Value:

- Calories: 264

- Protein: 5g
- Carbohydrates: 9g
- Fiber: 3g
- Fat: 24g

Recipe 37: Roasted Sweet Potatoes with Cinnamon

Prep Time: 10 minutes Cook Time: 25 minutes Serves: 4

Ingredients:

- 2 large sweet potatoes, peeled and diced
- 2 tbsp olive oil
- 1 tsp ground cinnamon
- Salt and pepper to taste
- Fresh thyme leaves for garnish

Directions:

1. Preheat the oven to 425°F (220°C).
2. In a bowl, toss diced sweet potatoes with olive oil, ground cinnamon, salt, and pepper.
3. Spread them on a baking sheet in a single layer.

4. Roast for 20-25 minutes, stirring once, until sweet potatoes are tender and caramelized.

5. Garnish with fresh thyme leaves before serving.

Nutritional Value:

- Calories: 168
- Protein: 2g
- Carbohydrates: 27g
- Fiber: 4g
- Fat: 7g

Recipe 38: Strawberry Spinach Salad

Prep Time: 10 minutes Serves: 4

Ingredients:

- 6 cups fresh baby spinach leaves
- 1 1/2 cups sliced strawberries
- 1/4 cup red onion, thinly sliced
- 1/4 cup chopped pecans, toasted
- 1/4 cup crumbled goat cheese
- Balsamic vinaigrette dressing

Directions:

1. In a large bowl, combine fresh baby spinach leaves, sliced strawberries, thinly sliced red onion, and toasted chopped pecans.

2. Drizzle with balsamic vinaigrette dressing and toss gently.

3. Sprinkle crumbled goat cheese on top before serving.

Nutritional Value:

- Calories: 143
- Protein: 3g
- Carbohydrates: 11g
- Fiber: 3g
- Fat: 10g

Recipe 39: Honey-Garlic Shrimp and Broccoli

Prep Time: 15 minutes Cook Time: 15 minutes Serves: 2

Ingredients:

- 16 large shrimp, peeled and deveined
- 2 cups broccoli florets
- 2 cloves garlic, minced

- 2 tbsp honey
- 2 tbsp low-sodium soy sauce
- 1 tbsp olive oil
- Salt and pepper to taste
- Sesame seeds for garnish

Directions:

1. In a bowl, whisk together minced garlic, honey, low-sodium soy sauce, olive oil, salt, and pepper.
2. Marinate shrimp in the mixture for 10 minutes.
3. Heat a skillet over medium-high heat. Add marinated shrimp and cook for 2-3 minutes per side until pink and opaque. Remove from the skillet.
4. In the same skillet, add broccoli florets and a splash of water. Cover and steam for 3-4 minutes until tender.
5. Return cooked shrimp to the skillet and toss with the broccoli.
6. Garnish with sesame seeds before serving.

Nutritional Value:

- Calories: 289

- Protein: 21g
- Carbohydrates: 27g
- Fiber: 4g
- Fat: 12g

Recipe 40: Quinoa and Chickpea Stuffed Bell Peppers

Prep Time: 20 minutes Cook Time: 45 minutes Serves: 4

Ingredients:

- 4 large bell peppers, any color
- 1 cup cooked quinoa
- 1 can (15 oz) chickpeas, drained and rinsed
- 1 cup diced tomatoes
- 1/2 cup chopped fresh parsley
- 1/2 cup crumbled feta cheese
- 1/2 tsp ground cumin
- Salt and pepper to taste
- Fresh mint leaves for garnish

Directions:

1. Preheat the oven to 375°F (190°C).

2. Cut the tops off the bell peppers and remove seeds and membranes.

3. In a bowl, mix cooked quinoa, chickpeas, diced tomatoes, chopped fresh parsley, crumbled feta cheese, ground cumin, salt, and pepper.

4. Stuff each bell pepper with the quinoa and chickpea mixture.

5. Place stuffed peppers in a baking dish and cover with foil.

6. Bake for 30 minutes, then remove foil and bake for an additional 15 minutes until peppers are tender.

7. Garnish with fresh mint leaves and serve.

Nutritional Value:

- Calories: 314
- Protein: 12g
- Carbohydrates: 51g
- Fiber: 11g
- Fat: 7g

Recipe 41: Mediterranean Orzo Salad

Prep Time: 15 minutes Serves: 4

Ingredients:

- 1 cup orzo pasta, cooked and cooled
- 1 cup cucumber, diced
- 1 cup cherry tomatoes, halved
- 1/2 cup Kalamata olives, pitted and sliced
- 1/2 cup crumbled feta cheese
- 1/4 cup red onion, finely chopped
- 2 tbsp fresh oregano, chopped
- Juice of 1 lemon
- 2 tbsp olive oil
- Salt and pepper to taste

Directions:

1. In a large bowl, combine cooked orzo pasta, diced cucumber, halved cherry tomatoes, sliced Kalamata olives, crumbled feta cheese, finely chopped red onion, and chopped fresh oregano.

2. In a separate bowl, whisk together lemon juice, olive oil, salt, and pepper.

3. Drizzle the dressing over the salad and toss gently.

4. Serve as a refreshing side dish.

Nutritional Value:

- Calories: 300
- Protein: 9g
- Carbohydrates: 39g
- Fiber: 4g
- Fat: 13g

Recipe 42: Grilled Lemon Garlic Asparagus

Prep Time: 10 minutes Cook Time: 10 minutes Serves: 4

Ingredients:

- 1 bunch asparagus, trimmed
- 2 tbsp olive oil
- Zest and juice of 1 lemon
- 2 cloves garlic, minced
- Salt and pepper to taste

- Grated Parmesan cheese for garnish (optional)

Directions:

1. Preheat the grill to medium-high heat.
2. In a bowl, toss trimmed asparagus with olive oil, lemon zest, lemon juice, minced garlic, salt, and pepper.
3. Grill asparagus for 5-7 minutes, turning occasionally, until tender and slightly charred.
4. Garnish with grated Parmesan cheese before serving if desired.

Nutritional Value:

- Calories: 63
- Protein: 2g
- Carbohydrates: 5g
- Fiber: 2g
- Fat: 4g

Recipe 43: Avocado Tomato Salad

Prep Time: 10 minutes Serves: 4

Ingredients:

- 2 avocados, diced

- 2 cups cherry tomatoes, halved
- 1/4 cup red onion, finely chopped
- 1/4 cup fresh cilantro, chopped
- Juice of 1 lime
- Salt and pepper to taste

Directions:

1. In a bowl, combine diced avocados, halved cherry tomatoes, finely chopped red onion, chopped fresh cilantro, and lime juice.
2. Season with salt and pepper, and gently toss to combine.
3. Serve as a flavorful side dish.

Nutritional Value:

- Calories: 182
- Protein: 2g
- Carbohydrates: 12g
- Fiber: 7g
- Fat: 15g

Recipe 44: Butternut Squash and Apple Soup

Prep Time: 15 minutes Cook Time: 30 minutes Serves: 4

Ingredients:

- 1 butternut squash, peeled, seeded, and diced
- 2 apples, peeled, cored, and diced
- 1 onion, chopped
- 2 cloves garlic, minced
- 4 cups vegetable broth
- 1/2 tsp ground cinnamon
- 1/4 tsp ground nutmeg
- Salt and pepper to taste
- Greek yogurt for garnish (optional)

Directions:

1. In a large pot, sauté chopped onions and minced garlic until softened.
2. Add diced butternut squash, diced apples, vegetable broth, ground cinnamon, ground nutmeg, salt, and pepper.

3. Bring to a boil, then reduce heat and simmer for 25-30 minutes, or until squash and apples are tender.

4. Use an immersion blender to puree the soup until smooth.

5. Garnish with a dollop of Greek yogurt if desired.

Nutritional Value:

- Calories: 153
- Protein: 2g
- Carbohydrates: 38g
- Fiber: 6g
- Fat

Recipe 45: Baked Lemon Herb Tilapia

Prep Time: 10 minutes Cook Time: 15 minutes Serves: 2

Ingredients:

- 2 tilapia fillets
- Zest and juice of 1 lemon
- 2 tbsp olive oil
- 1 tsp dried thyme

- 1/2 tsp dried rosemary
- Salt and pepper to taste
- Lemon wedges for garnish

Directions:

1. Preheat the oven to 375°F (190°C).
2. In a bowl, whisk together lemon zest, lemon juice, olive oil, dried thyme, dried rosemary, salt, and pepper.
3. Place tilapia fillets in a baking dish and drizzle with the lemon-herb mixture.
4. Bake for 12-15 minutes, or until fish flakes easily with a fork.
5. Garnish with lemon wedges before serving.

Nutritional Value:

- Calories: 196
- Protein: 23g
- Carbohydrates: 2g
- Fiber: 0g
- Fat: 11g

Recipe 46: Spinach and Mushroom Stuffed Acorn Squash

Prep Time: 20 minutes Cook Time: 45 minutes Serves: 4

Ingredients:

- 2 acorn squash, halved and seeds removed
- 2 cups fresh spinach leaves
- 1 cup mushrooms, sliced
- 1/2 cup grated Gruyere cheese
- 2 cloves garlic, minced
- 2 tbsp olive oil
- Salt and pepper to taste

Directions:

1. Preheat the oven to 375°F (190°C).
2. Brush the cut sides of the acorn squash with olive oil and season with salt and pepper.
3. Place squash halves, cut side down, on a baking sheet.
4. Roast for 35-40 minutes until the flesh is tender.
5. While the squash is roasting, sauté sliced mushrooms in a pan with minced garlic until tender.

6. Add fresh spinach to the pan and cook until wilted.

7. Remove from heat and stir in grated Gruyere cheese.

8. Stuff each acorn squash half with the spinach and mushroom mixture.

9. Return to the oven and bake for an additional 5-10 minutes until cheese is melted and bubbly.

Nutritional Value:

- Calories: 225
- Protein: 6g
- Carbohydrates: 37g
- Fiber: 6g
- Fat: 9g

Recipe 47: Lemon Rosemary Grilled Chicken

Prep Time: 15 minutes Cook Time: 15 minutes Serves: 4

Ingredients:

- 4 boneless, skinless chicken breasts
- Zest and juice of 1 lemon
- 2 tbsp olive oil

- 1 tbsp fresh rosemary, chopped
- 2 cloves garlic, minced
- Salt and pepper to taste
- Fresh rosemary sprigs for garnish

Directions:

1. In a bowl, whisk together lemon zest, lemon juice, olive oil, chopped fresh rosemary, minced garlic, salt, and pepper.
2. Marinate chicken breasts in the mixture for 10 minutes.
3. Preheat the grill to medium-high heat.
4. Grill chicken for about 6-7 minutes per side, or until cooked through.
5. Garnish with fresh rosemary sprigs before serving.

Nutritional Value:

- Calories: 215
- Protein: 27g
- Carbohydrates: 2g
- Fiber: 0g

- Fat: 11g

Recipe 48: Roasted Beet and Goat Cheese Salad

Prep Time: 15 minutes Cook Time: 45 minutes Serves: 4

Ingredients:

- 4 medium-sized beets, peeled and diced
- 4 cups mixed greens
- 1/2 cup crumbled goat cheese
- 1/4 cup walnuts, toasted and chopped
- Balsamic vinaigrette dressing

Directions:

1. Preheat the oven to 375°F (190°C).
2. Toss diced beets with a little olive oil, salt, and pepper.
3. Roast in the oven for 40-45 minutes until tender.
4. Let the beets cool slightly.
5. In a large salad bowl, combine mixed greens, roasted beets, crumbled goat cheese, and toasted chopped walnuts.
6. Drizzle with balsamic vinaigrette dressing and toss gently.

Nutritional Value:

- Calories: 225
- Protein: 8g
- Carbohydrates: 14g
- Fiber: 4g
- Fat: 16g

Recipe 49: Quinoa-Stuffed Portobello Mushrooms

Prep Time: 15 minutes Cook Time: 20 minutes Serves: 4

Ingredients:

- 4 large Portobello mushrooms, stems removed
- 1 cup cooked quinoa
- 1/2 cup diced red bell pepper
- 1/2 cup diced zucchini
- 1/4 cup grated Parmesan cheese
- 2 cloves garlic, minced
- 2 tbsp olive oil
- Salt and pepper to taste
- Fresh basil leaves for garnish

Directions:

1. Preheat the oven to 375°F (190°C).
2. Place Portobello mushrooms on a baking sheet, cap side down.
3. In a bowl, combine cooked quinoa, diced red bell pepper, diced zucchini, grated Parmesan cheese, minced garlic, olive oil, salt, and pepper.
4. Stuff each mushroom with the quinoa mixture.
5. Bake for 20 minutes until mushrooms are tender and filling is heated through.
6. Garnish with fresh basil leaves before serving.

Nutritional Value:

- Calories: 207
- Protein: 7g
- Carbohydrates: 26g
- Fiber: 4g
- Fat: 9g

Recipe 50: Grilled Vegetable Platter with Hummus

Prep Time: 15 minutes Cook Time: 10 minutes Serves: 4

Ingredients:

- 2 zucchinis, sliced lengthwise
- 2 bell peppers (red and yellow), quartered
- 1 red onion, cut into wedges
- 2 tbsp olive oil
- Salt and pepper to taste
- Hummus for dipping

Directions:

1. Preheat the grill to medium-high heat.
2. Toss zucchini slices, bell pepper quarters, and red onion wedges with olive oil, salt, and pepper.
3. Grill the vegetables for 4-5 minutes per side, or until they have grill marks and are tender.
4. Arrange grilled vegetables on a platter and serve with hummus for dipping.

Nutritional Value:

- Calories: 133

- Protein: 3g
- Carbohydrates: 10g
- Fiber: 3g
- Fat: 10g

CONCLUSION

As we reach the conclusion of the "Fibroid-Shrinking Recipes Cookbook," we want to express our sincere hope that this collection of recipes has not only filled your kitchen with delicious flavors but also filled your heart with a sense of empowerment and well-being.

Your health journey is a personal one, and we believe that what you eat can be a transformative force for good. By choosing to embrace these fibroid-shrinking recipes, you've taken a positive step toward nurturing your body and supporting your overall health. Whether you are actively managing fibroids or simply seeking to lead a healthier life, every meal you prepare from these pages is a gift to yourself.

We encourage you to continue exploring the world of wholesome and nutrient-rich foods, to listen to your body, and to savor each bite with mindfulness and gratitude. Your well-being is worth the investment of time and care, and we trust that these recipes have provided you with the tools and inspiration to make healthier choices.

Remember that your health journey is unique, and it's okay to seek guidance from healthcare professionals who can provide tailored advice and support. Combine their expertise with the knowledge and delicious recipes you've discovered in this cookbook, and you'll be well-equipped to make informed decisions about your dietary choices.

We want to extend our heartfelt thanks for joining us on this culinary adventure. We hope that these recipes have become more than just ingredients and instructions—they are an integral part of your path to wellness, vitality, and self-care.

May the flavors and nourishment you've experienced within these pages continue to bring you joy, strength, and a profound sense of well-being. Here's to a future filled with vibrant health, delicious meals, and the knowledge that you have the power to support your body's journey toward balance and vitality.

Thank you for allowing us to be a part of your health and wellness journey. Cheers to a healthier, happier you!

Printed in Great Britain
by Amazon